GETTING OLDER

AND

ENJOYING IT!

Lura Zerick

ISBN 0-7414-2099-6

Published by:

INFINITY
PUBLISHING.COM

1094 New Dehaven Street, Suite 100
West Conshohocken, PA 19428-2713
Info@buybooksontheweb.com
www.buybooksontheweb.com
Toll-free (877) BUY BOOK
Local Phone (610) 941-9999
Fax (610) 941-9959

Printed in the United States of America

Printed on Recycled Paper

Published July 2004

DEDICATED TO SENIORS EVERYWHERE

AND IN MEMORY OF

A COUSIN,

LIFETIME FRIEND AND CLASSMATE:

JUANITA SPEARS MESSER

AND TO SPECIAL FRIENDS:

BOBBIE, CAROLYN, DORIS,
GIANGI, JACKIE AND JANET

New grandson, little Eddie, wasn't included in
the last book; he is listed in this one

DISCLAIMER

This book is written to provide information on how to have a more fulfilling and rewarding life as a senior citizen. Neither the author or publisher are engaged in rendering any form of professional services. If expert assistance is required, the services of a competent professional should be sought.

Every effort has been made to make this book as complete and accurate as possible. This text should be used only as a general guide and not as the ultimate source for living.

My goal is to educate as well as entertain; that is why I have sprinkled a few humorous items so that you, the reader, might enjoy a few chuckles as you identify with other seniors in this sometimes entertaining experience we call life. Remember that laughter is probably as good a medicine as we will find. Try it!

Lura Spears Zerick

TOPICS

BE PROUD OF YOUR AGE!

Getting older is a subject that most don't want to talk about; if we don't discuss it, maybe it will go away. Wrong! Age is a fact of life, regardless of where we are in the numbers game. Why do so many want to stay twenty or thirty or forty? Just as each season has its' own beauty, so does each year or each decade. We can learn to look forward to the coming years instead of dreading them.

Up to our early teens, we are children playing grown up. We can't wait to be an adult; we don't think of the bigger decisions or responsibility we will have. Most children are thinking of the freedom they will have, naively thinking that is the key to living.

For many of us, twenty was a time of rash decisions which might have brought painful consequences. When we arrive at the point of being a legal adult, we often refuse to face any responsibility and often make worse decisions. These might bring other results and we find ourselves on the merry-go-round of life and sometimes we never get off of it. Life is not a race to see who can get there first. We already are. We can relax about getting older every year.

We waste so much time as we plan ahead on what we will or won't do. We might not have tomorrow; none of us can be certain. We spend the present making plans for the future. When we have those plans set in out minds, we waste today as we regret yesterday. We throw the time away as if we don't want or need it!.

When we have rough patches in our lives, as all of us do, we continue to waste today as we dread tomorrow and are often disgusted by the past. Can we gain anything by that attitude? We can fret until we turn purple and nothing will change. The situation won't get better, we won't grow another inch taller and we still have to face the consequences of our actions.

With all these decisions, why not decide to learn more about enjoying life in the now? As one guy stated, "If I wake up, it's a good day." We are given the gift of each day and we whine and moan all the way through it! Have we really become adults or are we acting like children?

When we are planning a vacation trip we decide where we are going, where we will stay and what we will do when we get there. Do we decide somewhere along the line that we don't want to finish the trip? Do we want to enjoy only the beginning and maybe the middle of the journey? Isn't that silly! Wouldn't we laugh if someone suggested that for our vacation? Yet we seem to prefer that when it refers to life or our getting older.

As we travel on our own pathway of life, do we prefer the beginning and the middle of this learning experience? The end of our trip can be pleasant, enjoyable, fun, rewarding, challenging, fulfilling and more. Why would we want to miss all that? These days can be more wonderful than our earlier ones. Our attitudes determine the results. If we think negative, so will our days be.

When we learn to appreciate life for what it is, a gift given to us to open and explore, then we can be grateful for each day. We don't stop living the moment we get on Medicare! Truthfully, the best might be yet to come! Retirement from one job might mean the beginning of another career.

Instead of moping through each day, we should treat those hours as if we can't bear to lose them! That is exactly what we often do – not only lose them but actually throw them away! We know that we won't ever be able to pick them up again tomorrow; only later will we realize what that mistake has cost us.

We could take an idea from a clock; keep ticking day after day, never trying to rush or slow anything but just living the moment. When we learn to do that, life will be more fulfilling and rewarding. We won't fret about the past or the future, but simply enjoy the present regardless of age. The word present can have the same meaning as the word gift and that is actually what we have: the gift of life, given to us from God.

A BICYCLE AT LAST!

I have longed for a bicycle all my life! After becoming an adult, I could have bought one but I was busy raising my five children. Besides, I didn't have confidence of staying on it very long. I didn't want to fall off in front of the kids! After all, I've spent a total of less than one hour on a bike; most of this time spent in trying to get the hang of it. Finally, as a senior citizen, it looks like I will be getting a bike, as per doctor's orders; he told me to start riding a bike for my exercise.

When I was around eight years old I spent many days trying to build a bicycle, certain that I could get a working model together. Any advice I needed could come from my older and wiser brother. Some of my materials included two old car tires, a hammer, a few nails and a small board for a seat. Oh, the imagination of a child is wonderful! I finally gave up on this idea and adjusted to never having a bike. Also, my brother was too busy to help on this important project. None of my friends had bikes either, which was why I couldn't get more experience in riding one.

After all these years, my dream might come true but it won't really be a bicycle. Actually, it will be a tricycle but in my eyes it will be a realized goal. It doesn't matter that it will be a three-wheeler, the kind often seen whizzing around senior communities. Who cares? To me it will be my dream bicycle. Maybe it won't be "whizzing around" but it will be moving on wheels with ME sitting on the seat!

Though I have enjoyed walking distances most of my life, changes in my knees have almost ruled that pleasure out. At age 73, after dancing millions of miles and walking numerous country roads, I will be enjoying my bicycle, uh, tricycle, as often as possible. I expect to continue driving my car, even the 500 miles to my other home, but probably not as often as in the past. I'm sure it will take a longer time as I make more stops along the way. I will still make it in one day – up to the woods and the whippowills. These are more calming than the sirens of my city home.

While this probably will slow my activities a bit, I refuse to let this get me down. I look at it as an opportunity to be 'up and away'. I'm so glad that I'm getting my bicycle at last! If I can turn loose with one hand, I'll wave!

LEARNING TO ENJOY
OUR LATER YEARS

Some spend their days, sometimes lives, regretting the past, hating the present and dreading the future. Many of us have been there. Though it takes awhile before we learn to appreciate the NOW, we must realize that now is all we have.

We waste years wanting to undo the past; the present is difficult and the future looks bleak. When we realize that life is too short to throw away, we will be grateful for the gift of each day. Our new attitude will change our lives.

We have to let go of the past – there is nothing we can do about it. Now we have the time to reach for the dreams we had years ago. We will be amazed at our success; being confident still seems a new experience. We can do things that we would have avoided in the past, though we might have wanted to do them. We might have let the fear of failure keep us from even trying.

If we did try, we often failed because we thought we would. Never accomplishing anything is really to fail. It is much better to try and fail than never to have tried. We could spend the rest of our lives wondering if we might have been successful.

Isn't it better to know? If we fail at one thing, we simply go on to the next item on the list. We might not win every time but that is no reason to give up. When we think we can succeed, we usually do. The boost to our confidence is more than can be expressed.

We are no longer the zeros that we saw years ago; we are older people who appreciate our God-given abilities. We are aware that life is too precious to waste; now we can enjoy those things we are capable of doing. We like where we are and who we are. Something wonderful could happen today! We enjoy being parents, grandparents as well as great grandparents but we know that we are also people who can accomplish a lot.

Our children are adults and busy with their children. We can look at the "empty nest" as our opportunities to reach for the goals we had when we were young. It is extremely satisfying to know that we might still contribute to the lives of others.

It is very important that we learn to laugh. Instead of walking around with a frown, let's begin to smile in gratitude for just being alive. Amazingly, when we smile our faces are transformed. Our expressions can draw others to us or turn them away. Do YOU like to be around someone who always wears a sour look? Be honest; you usually look for another direction to avoid them, right?

Those who are upbeat and enthusiastic about life usually draw us to them. We want a taste of their joy in living, though we might never admit such a thing. They appear to be stronger personalities as compared to our feeling like wimps. We long to be like them but have no inkling of how or where to begin.

One of the first steps is to learn that our lives are a gift from God. We didn't just happen to be here all of a sudden; there is a purpose for each life. Look at the abilities you have been given; have you used them? Think about what you enjoy doing most. It might be that your purpose will use that ability. If it doesn't, you will have the ability to learn what ever you need to fulfill that purpose. Don't hang back in the shadows, go for it!

OBSERVATIONS OF A SENIOR

I like being older; I enjoy being more successful than when I was young. I enjoy having more wisdom than in the past. I like being capable of doing many things. I look forward to each day. What I don't like is being overlooked as if I'm not there.

It happens all the time. When others look at me, they see a 5'6" fairly slender lady with silver hair and green eyes. My hair is silver by choice; I happen to like it! I was a blonde most of my life but now I just want to be ME. I'm not trying to be young again – who in their right mind would want that? Yes, I'm older but I'm still me! I tell the hairdresser that I'm not there for her to make me look young; just make me a sharp looking old lady! Who says I can't look good because I'm old? YOU? Duh!

Many think they see a sweet little great-granny who doesn't know much. I am a sweet little great-granny (most of the time) but I'm also much more. Read my lips: I'm not a has-been; I still am. I refuse to let life drag me down ever again. It almost whipped me in earlier years but I find that I'm like a boomerang – I keep coming back! I'm not a quitter anymore. I'm a survivor and intend to stay one!

My five are grown-up and scattered; my 13 grandchildren are unusually intelligent, talented and beautiful; my two great-grands show wonderful promise. I am now free to do my thing, which definitely is not lying around in my robe watching the soaps. I've already lived most of those situations; I should be writing them!

What I am writing, and getting published, are songs, articles and books. I can tell you, it is much better than dreading the day and wishing I could be some place else. It is much better than the feeling of failure that crushed me most of my life. What I had to learn, aside from what the hard knocks taught me, was to change my ATTITUDE!

I though I was a failure so I was. Now I know I'm not and I succeed! It's almost that simple! When my failures beat me down (along with many fists, feet and words), I was convinced that I had no worth; I was a total failure. I was, as long as I thought that way.

Once I remembered that I am an intelligent and capable person and gained the confidence of that fact, I was on my way. I can tell you, I'm traveling down this road until my last breath. I'm hoping many of you will join me and wake up to this new world of possibilities. Don't dismiss me as being nothing worth noticing. I'm into accomplishment and don't have time to waste with those who decide to throw their lives away. I'm using the talents that God gave me and I always ask Him to direct me. I want to be the one He sees in me.

Under my 73-year-old heart is a person than can and will realize her dream. I use my experiences and wisdom to do things that many never consider.

Why? Because they don't believe they can! The difference is that I do!

Yes, I might forget what I had for supper last night but I can still name the major bones of the body that I learned when I was 12. I always say that I never forget anything but occasionally things might slip from my mind.

What I'm trying to say is don't dismiss me as if I'm a nothing because I am a senior citizen. Listen up, you might learn something! I fought and won the battle of being somebody and I refuse to allow anyone to change that fact. Having God's everlasting love even makes me someone special.

Did YOU let go of a goal because you thought you couldn't reach it? What might YOU be able to do when you decide you can? Do it now; it's never too late to learn. You can dream big as easily as you can dream small. If you fail, just go on to the next dream. It's your decision and your future depends on your response.

HELP! I'M BEING CHASED
BY WRINKLES!

"Hey, wait a minute!" I swung back toward the mirror I'd been walking past. I had glanced something I hadn't seen before. The left side of my face was covered with wrinkles! I'm serious! The right side looked the same as always but the left side appeared to be one wide bunch of wrinkles! Unbelievable! I'm sure those weren't there yesterday!

As I stared at my face I realized that I was there at last. I was turning into an old person right before my eyes! I am 73, but I've never felt old; I've always had the energy and attitude of someone much younger. I've never worried about my age – it's just another thing we have no control over. We are what we are and I accept that. Those who are vain about their age just make me chuckle. They are fighting a losing battle and don't even realize it. Would they prefer the alternative?

So what if I'm getting old? I am still breathing and I have things to do and age has nothing to do with it. I'm still me so what's a few more wrinkles? Didn't someone once say that wrinkles give 'character' to a face? I was seeing character eye to eye; there was no double about it! Those wrinkles are on my face, though, not my brain.

I already knew that when I smile, most of the facial wrinkles practically disappear! In that moment, while considering the newer wrinkles I had seen, I knew it would be necessary to have a bigger smile. Hello, world – I might have a few wrinkles but that won't stop me. I've learned that my attitude determines whether or not I succeed.

It will take more than a bunch of wrinkles to slow me down. I'm coming through and I have things to do – and I won't forget to smile!

AGE IS A STATE OF MIND

With mischief in her eye, one of my sisters told me that when you get old, you can get away with anything. I've been trying to learn if I'm there yet. Truthfully, I don't want to be young again, though in part of my mind, I still am. I feel much younger now, at 73, than when I was in my 20s or 30s; that's when I felt old. It seems only months ago that my five were small but I realize that time has flown. I am reminded how short life really is. I intend to enjoy and appreciate the gift of each day; I won't have the opportunity of it again.

I went through the 'material things' phase years ago and I learned a few things. I know that a big, beautiful home can become just a house. Diamonds don't mean much amid constant turmoil. I don't try to impress anyone. Traumatic experiences have helped me become strong; I became a survivor instead of a quitter. I'm grateful and appreciate my physical and mental health.

I don't need anyone's permission to wear whatever I prefer. I note that many wear what looks like what everyone else is wearing. I like to be ME: I don't try to imitate anyone and certainly don't want to meet myself walking down the street. I prefer to have a 'style' of my own.

I choose what looks good on me, not what someone else prefers. I don't care if it it's not what others are wearing; I don't want to look like anyone else. You'd have to use force to make me wear some of the 'fashionable' clothes I see when I window shop. I wear my hair short, so it won't drag my face downward – who needs that? Yes, I have wrinkles, so what? When I smile you see fewer of them. You don't believe me? Go smile in the mirror and see if I'm not right! I enjoy the expressions of the hairdresser when I tell her that I'm not there for her to make me look young. She probably thinks I'm a little strange but who cares?

It took a long time for me to get here. I wasted years, cried gallons of tears and spent a lot of money trying to please others. I finally realized that was impossible so I decided that I would please myself and in the process, try to please my Heavenly Father. Believe me, this is much more fun! I like every day now, instead of dreading that someone might remind me of what I've done wrong.

I'm reaching for, and attaining, goals that others would have laughed at in the past. So what? It doesn't matter what others say. I make my decisions; if I make the wrong one, I'm the one who suffers the consequences. I have learned a lot from wrong decisions. These have helped me grow.

My dreams can come true if I pursue them. It takes effort and energy, plus determination, but I can handle that. With God's help I have come from despair to success. When I was in deep depression, no one reminded me that I was an intelligent person who'd had many dreams. I thought that I was a failure, so I was. I allowed others to convince me that I was a total flop, period. Wrong!

When I decided I was someone who could succeed, I did. No one else is responsible for my happiness; I am. These days I expect little from others and a lot from myself. I like where I am and WHO I AM. It's terrific to look forward to each day, knowing something wonderful might happen. When it does, I'm not surprised, only grateful.

Do I sound rebellious? Not at all; I simply decided that I would be the one to say whether or not I was a failure. Since I made that decision, life has been full of challenge. How do I know I won't succeed unless I try? I'd rather try and fail than never to have tried and have the feeling that brings.

Success means different things to different people. I believe that one is a success when he or she learns to appreciate God-given abilities as well as the gift of life. Financial success is terrific, but there are many ways to be rich.

If you want to join me, then dig up your old dreams and grab onto one or more. You can be and do what you wanted years ago. Maybe the raising of your children intervened for awhile but they are no longer at home. What do you have to lose? You have time on your hands; you have to do something. Success doesn't have an age limit; this could be your time. Neither you nor I are responsible for anyone's success except our own.

If you have no dream to reach for, then you might spend your spare hours helping others. There are hundreds of fields that need volunteers and numerous ways to help others. You can know the joy and satisfaction that you have been a blessing to someone less fortunate than you. It is a great feeling, one that has no price. What can you do to help? Look into this possibility; you won't regret it.

I have learned to enjoy my solitude; it is during my quiet times that I learn how to live, whatever my age. I can also review, and be grateful for, all my blessings. It could be that the best is yet to come! Living with expectation is great!

THINK SUCCESS,
REGARDLESS OF AGE

It might be that you are in your sixties or seventies or older and you don't believe that you have been a success at anything. This might even be true but do you realize how much your attitude determines whether or not you succeed? It has everything to do with the outcome. First of all, if you are depending on God for your guidance and help, you are already on the road to success. I honestly believe that we must look to Him to lead us in our purpose. When we travel on our own road we can be fairly certain of failure because we are moving on our plans for us. That usually doesn't work and if it does we might have more heartbreak and disappointment coming at us.

I have been down the road I chose and I messed up more than ever. I have learned to ask for literal permission before I choose which path to take. If we don't do this, we will have opportunities to grow even more and the outcome might not be pleasant.

Yes, we can have dozens of ideas to work on but all of them are not for us. We need to learn which idea we should put our energy and effort in as we strive for a positive outcome.

If you think failure, it is certain that you will fail. If you begin something with the sense that you can't do it, you probably won't. Why even start if you believe you will fail? If you don't know how to do whatever is necessary for the success of some venture, then learn! If you give your time to a project, give it your best and do it well! Don't have the attitude that you can stumble through this and go on to the next step. Take pride in whatever you do; the results of your actions will follow you.

Whatever you're doing, how does this fit in with the purpose of your life? Do you know the reason you are living? What is your dream? What do you enjoy doing most and how might that coincide with your life's purpose? How many know their purpose and have acted accordingly? I don't believe that God has made a plan for your life that includes something you hate to do! Obviously, everything would work together better if this involves something that you enjoy doing.

For those who are still wondering what their purpose is, follow through in your thoughts with what you have a passion for. What is it that you are burning to do? What would you like to be a part in changing? What means so much to you that you are fired up every time you think about it? Complete these thoughts and you might have found the reason you are living. Don't you find this exciting?

In the middle of all this is your dream…the dream that has hovered around in your head for years. What is yours? It's okay to talk about it, bring it out for yourself and others to see. Look at it, talk about it. Can it become a reality? YOU are the only one who can answer that question because you are the one who will give the energy and effort to make it real. You can let others stop you if you aren't sure what you want. Only your determination can bring success and this will happen only if you plan each day around your goal.

Remember, you are not to neglect other important things in order to succeed. Your family's needs and your mate are not to be ignored during your quest. At no time should they be hungry or in dirty clothes so you might pursue your objective. If you are the husband, then you also know that you still are to provide for your family. To ignore their needs would show your worth as a husband and father.

Too many run after success in some venture, never realizing that this is not the path they should take. They might even have the wrong goal. This is why it is important that we seek wisdom and guidance from God instead of jumping out on our own. Believe me, relying on ourselves will bring more despair and disappointment than you can imagine.

You don't want to judge the present effort by another incident in your life where you didn't succeed. This is easy to do and you will fall into that trap if you aren't careful. An effort of the past has nothing to do with now. What you do in the present will certainly tell you what you can expect in the future. It is the future we are planning on, isn't it? So many waste the present because of the past and in doing this they ensure that there is little future. You might have a future but it will be as empty as those other years. Why not do what you can to make the present and future more wonderful?

You must focus on your plans; things don't just fall into place. Someone must carefully make plans that will bring success. If you have stood around all your life, waiting for someone else to bring out the plans, then you probably are drowning in the sense of disappointment and failure.

You are the plan-maker! You must know what you want to accomplish; you can't hang out in someone else's dream. Get your own dream. Whatever you plan to do, keep your attitude on being a victor and you will be a winner. Don't allow the sense of failure to corrupt your thoughts but think success. One of the greatest things you will ever learn is that YOU control your thoughts! This can and will make a tremendous difference in how you look at life, people and goals. You don't have to be disillusioned or swim around in failure. Take the next step and go on. Every journey is one step after the other. You can get to the destination of success if you just keep walking. This is the way to accomplishment and in being all you can be.

In order to do whatever you have chosen, you will learn to use your time effectively. Don't waste any precious minutes or seconds gossiping on the phone; this will only drag you further from your goal. You are already in the winter of your life, why would you throw away the gift of hours that are given each day? Think about these things each time you waver in making a decision on what to do next. Ask whether it will deter you or help you to accomplish your goal more quickly? Remember, most good goals are not reached within hours. Don't lessen the importance of your aim by doing silly things that will supposedly help you get there faster. Whatever your venture is, take your time and do it well. You don't want to look back and say, if only I had done so and so. Go slow and keep in mind that this is not a life or death matter. If it is meant for you to succeed, you will. If not, then it possibly was not the thing for you to do.

Your self-image hangs in the balance. You must have the confidence to gain your goals; don't let a negative thought throw you for a loop. Keep your dream in the foremost of your thoughts but make certain that it is the right dream. Your dream doesn't have to be a world shaking idea. Small dreams are important too. The size of your dream is up to you. It will be your efforts that make your dream come true. Whatever it is, stay with it until you are happy with the positive results.

If you can't seem to gain the self confidence for your dream, look at the fact that you are really just like most others. Do you think God would give one person the ability to do something and not another? Certainly not! Each of us is capable of doing something really well and that includes you! Remember that God is not a respecter of persons. Someone who is prettier or more wealthy than you doesn't have any better ability than you do. Have faith in your own abilities and use those God-given talents to do whatever you believe is your purpose in life.

Write those plans down; this will help you remember your goal. At our age, it is easy to forget where we want to go in life. A stumbling block can carry us around the block several times. We must learn to use these obstacles as stepping stones to the next rung on our ladder of dream realization.

Whatever you do, don't let the fact that you are a senior citizen stop you from reaching for a dream! As long as your mind is clear you can use it in many ways. Do it! Read as much as possible. Do those crossword puzzles. Find those words on a page of scrambled letters. Do everything that will help to keep you sharp and aware. Wouldn't you rather have a sense of accomplishment rather than sitting there waiting for the end of your life to happen? Don't waste these days you've been given. If possible, write someone a note. Pray for a loved one. Forgive those who have hurt you and throw away that grudge you've been carrying. Something like that will stop you in your tracks because you are using your energy on getting revenge instead of working toward your goal. Close that door and go forward. Don't allow someone else to determine whether you succeed in your undertaking.

Remember, your attitude is so important; age has little or nothing to do with it. Believe in yourself and your abilities and you will most likely reach your goal with a smile on your face. It is up to you. If this dream is important to you then make sure you continue to tell yourself "I know I can, I know I can, I know I can!" Don't just think it; do it!

I'M OLD ONLY ON THE OUTSIDE!

Most of us have heard that when several people see the same thing, each has a different version of what has been seen. That's also true in another area of life. Take me. When others see me moving around, they see an old lady carefully making her way across the room. Many dismiss me as just another senior creeping around, probably looking for another bingo game. Wrong! What they don't see is a well organized lady on the way to my next activity. You see, I'm old only on the outside.

Inside, my mind is alert to new ideas not only to write about but also ways to help others have a more fulfilling life. Of course, all that activity helps me to have a better life too. Now that is living! Anyway, I'm not really creeping around, I'm moving at my usual brisk pace (right?), sometimes an actual strut. You didn't know that a seventy-something can strut? All things are possible in the mind's eye. We think we're strutting, confident in the abilities we are using for mankind. That's not a true statement; we know that many men already know everything. Females seem to be more open to new ideas; they will listen and learn how to accomplish another success. They can usually put painful pasts behind them and go on to better and happier times. That is a special talent which moves us from one point to another, taking us from creeping around the halls of life to a strut that almost dares any obstacle to knock us down again. (Men, I'm just joking; you have great potential.)

Many aren't aware that seniors are still people. They consider that we are over, finished, done. Not so! We have danced a million miles, many of us still able to move pretty well when given the chance. We can still get up and sing, not only carrying the tune but also getting a lot of applause. No, it wasn't because we got to the end of the song! Many of us can whip up goodies that make others beg for more. It's not over 'til it's over, so stop acting like we're not there!

A special friend laughs as she reminds me that while others might think we are has-beens, just remember where we have been! She's right! We have lived life to the fullest, experiencing joy and pain in unequal amounts. It seemed like there was more pain, but as we found our resilient selves, we bounced back to enjoy life as it was meant to be.

Yeah, well, I'm still bouncing around; it just looks like I'm barely moving. In my mind I can still do those fancy jazz steps, sing that snappy song and even get across the street safely! I go roaring down the Interstate, intent on getting to my destination 500 miles away. I will admit that some of those pokey drivers get on my nerves but I simply pass them and go on my way. Maybe they're not going far but I am. I will be on time for that booksigning, speaking engagement, newspaper interview or television guest spot. Yeah! I enjoy all of those! Do you think I would consider changing these wonderful days for those years when I cried day and night? Talk about failing memory! I cried so long that I forgot what I was crying about!

Maybe I'm not creepy-crawling because I realize that time is getting shorter; I have to accomplish what I can while I can! I'll never go back to that failure mode; I'm out of there for good! Like the little engine that could, my motto now is "I think I can, I think I can!" So I do!

You might believe that I'm an old lady moving slowly through life but in reality I'm a high-stepping dame on my way to somewhere and having the time of my life! Why don't you join me?

SENIOR COMMUNITIES
AND RETIREMENT HOMES

These unique communities are found in most states, but especially in Florida and other sunny places that might bring older people to a warmer climate. In comparison with small villages, these are planned to fill every need of the senior citizen. These senior communities vary with availability in rentals and/or buying their own house or apartment. Often rentals can be shared with friends to help cover the costs.

Whatever their needs are, seniors can find the answer in the communities which are designed and planned to meet these needs. First of all, apartments or villas can be found with one or two bedrooms. The kitchens are fully equipped for those who enjoy cooking. In the larger communities, they can choose to take their meals in large dining rooms with others. Their 'homes' include walk-in closets, screened patios or balconies, walk-in showers, individual heat/air controls, smoke and fire detectors and various other choices.

Many of these communities offer rehabilitation services with in-house care and/or service. This helps to give their clients more independent and productive lives which contribute to the assurance that they are not a "burden" on their families.

Other specific offerings are a beauty and barber shop, valet laundry services, pets are often allowed and assisted living is available. These communities offer an uplifting atmosphere and blend their choices to compliment their lifestyle.

Amenities often include elegant dining rooms which serve two meals each day, Monday through Saturday, with Sunday brunch. Weekly housekeeping services are available. Along with the valet laundry services, flat laundry service is available. If the seniors choose, they can use the laundry facilities and do their own, if their health permits.

Scheduled transportation is available for those who don't or prefer not to drive. These destinations might include trips to the supermarket, public libraries, shopping, special entertainment or whatever else is necessary to make their lives better. Usually there is a small library in the clubhouse, readily available to those living there.

Most of the 'villages' offer 24-hour monitored security as well as health and safety emergency service. For those interested in arts and crafts there is a room where they can meet, have shows, work on their projects and generally share. Sometimes there is a 'thrift' store, offering items that some don't need to those who do. This can be one of the fun things for those who love a bargain.

For the exercise minded, there is usually a gym available at all hours, plus regular exercise programs for those who want to join a group. A heated swimming pool is there for the using as well as regular pool exercise. Games which offer another kind of exercise are shuffleboard or horseshoes. Some communities have putting greens for those who enjoy golf. Larger places have a golf course.

Card/dice games are numerous, including bunco, poker, rummy, scrabble, bridge, cribbage and pinochle. A card room is usually designated for these activities.

A larger social entertainment room for special events is available; these might include dances or parties, musical programs or specific speakers.

A barbeque pit, along with picnic tables, is available for the asking for family-get-togethers or other events. Some prefer this type of socializing to going out to a restaurant; the informality appeals to many.

SENIOR CARE

Many personal needs make up those which are available in several communities. These might include letter writing, light housekeeping, mailing bills or letters, arranging appointments and/or appointment reminders, help in paying bills, assistance in grooming or bathing, changing linen, bathroom cleanup, communications with family, meal planning/preparation/cleanup, maintenance scheduling, errand running, medication reminders, nutritional assessments, checking food freshness, dusting furniture, escorts on walks or trips to the beauty/barber shops, going out to lunch, grocery shopping, doing laundry or ironing, hurricane preparedness (if necessary), incidental transportation, organizing closets/drawers, sorting or answering mail, taking garbage out or vacuuming carpets. These services help seniors to remain independent in the familiar surroundings of their own home.

Anything not listed might also be available, according to their needs. Of course, there are thousands of seniors who are able to do all these things. Those who are mobile can and do get out and are active in outside programs. Some are able to work either full or part time, giving them a special outside interest. Many are involved in volunteer organizations, giving their abilities and experience to help others. Some are involved in the various kinds of ministries that help others grow spiritually. Some are available for counseling in different fields of employment. Their minds are still sharp and they use this wisdom for the good of others. One who has worked in a specific field can certainly advise one who wants to enter that field. Some of the pointers they give might save the younger person from making many mistakes over the coming years.

Experience is a great teacher, but we are wise when we learn from the experience of others. It is often much easier than having to learn through our own. Some are a little hard-headed, and are going their own way no matter what happens. Usually, a lot happens from these decisions and it is often bad.

HEALTH CARE

Health care is an important subject for seniors. After the age of 65 they are on Medicare but a supplement is necessary to cut the expense of illness. The cost of medicines soar, often costing hundreds of dollars each month for those who cannot afford these astronomical prices. They have no choice; they must have the medication even if this affects how often they eat. Many have a real problem of meeting their needs in all the areas that are too expensive for them. Too often they are put on more and more medication, making the total of daily pills rise to an alarming number. Some doctors add more pills with every office visit, placing the seniors in a sometimes dangerous position. They are afraid not to take the medications, yet the mixture of many medicines can be life-threatening.

Doctors want to know which medications a patient is presently taking, yet later during an office visit, they ask again, not remembering that these should be listed in the chart of the patient. With the number of patients served each day, there is no way a doctor can remember all the medications taken. It should be there in black and white for their reference when necessary.

Patients should note the side effects of each medicine for these can sometimes be worse than the original illness. Too, there is often the situation of being allergic to certain medications, which can bring greater pain and/or sickness to the patient.

Regarding the costs of drugs, many were eased financially in this situation with the availability of their medicines from Canada, with a base of operations in the United States. One such facility is located in Scottsdale, Arizona. They are celebrating their business of helping seniors and boasts of an impressive national customer base of thousands.

The Canadian lower prices and government approved medications, paid in U.S. funds, contribute to this success. Seniors often have limited incomes at the time when they need more medications. Many insurance companies are restrictive and often limit drug payments. Brand name drugs are excluded and these companies demand higher co-pays; sometimes they simply abolish existing drug coverage.

The services offered by the U.S. based Canadian company are ideal as they save thousands of dollars for the numerous seniors who use them.

This company, called Prescription Drugs Canada, is not an internet pharmacy; they are a U.S. company, following U.S. rules and regulations and drugs are paid for in U.S. currency. Other Canadian or Mexican internet companies are less strict. PDC has the interests of their patients in mind and tries to give them the security they want and need. They also provide telephone and walk-in customer service in Spanish and have a toll-free number available, 1-866-797-4337. They offer a money saving, secure, safe alternative that is more and more popular. Their website is www.pdcllp.com and offer any information that will help their customers. A toll-free phone number for English is 1-888-794-5377.

I'm sure there are other Canadian-priced pharmacies available but I have no information on these. As seniors, we are to find the best deal and still get the medications ordered by our doctors. When we can save money, that's great.

Of course, doctors are available from every field of medicine. Needs of seniors vary and it is necessary to have an expert in that area.

WANT SOMETHING DONE?
ASK A SENIOR!

Seniors are often the most dependable age group. Many who commit to do something might slide right on by; younger people often have their thoughts on other things and they can't be bothered. People in the senior citizen group are some of the most dependable when something needs to be done!

One 70-something professional stated that she far preferred a senior for her secretary rather than younger people. She gave the pros and cons, citing the reasons for her preference. Older women are more dependable, more likely to be at work when expected. They are often more loyal and trustworthy with the details of the office. They usually know how to solve simple negative situations.

Whereas, younger women might use any reason or excuse not to come to work. Sometimes they aren't concerned about what is needed at the office, only that they couldn't be there. Their children might be sick, or whatever, and this is a legitimate reason, but not helpful to a busy office.

Many churches and other organizations are held together by older men and women. Certainly senior males often make a contribution with their efforts and energy. Some groups might be run entirely by older men; they know what they want to accomplish and how to attain their goals. Sometimes younger men might be influenced by either their own needs and wants or by others. It is disappointing to have complete plans fall apart at the last moment because someone didn't care.

The workplace is filled with people over 55. Many seem in their prime of life, while others that same age might have little or no ambition to accomplish anything. Some of these might have followed their parents in the 'accomplish little' way of life. Others are still full of enthusiasm and eager to see what can be done. Age means nothing to these; they are only aware of the next thing they want to get done. They are a delight to be around; their eagerness often rubs off onto others. No one knows how this works, only that it does.

Some, young or old, simply go to their jobs day in and day out, never enjoying a moment of their day. They might have chosen the wrong career for various reasons. Many choose their profession because of the money they will make; they forget to ask themselves whether they will like doing that particular job. Money is a contributing factor but not the most important one. A job that we can enjoy, even with less pay, is much better than one that pays a lot more, but we hate to go to work.

When they choose something they will enjoy doing, they are far ahead of the game. Life will be happier; they will have a true feeling of accomplishment, which is a reward in itself. When will they learn that if they have a job they hate, that they will never be happy there, regardless of the money they make. What good is it when you pay your funds out for health problems, or spend your extra money on things that might bring you down? Being miserable on the job can bring many disasters into one's life. Having a job they will enjoy will make the difference between living and existing.

Just imagine something you would hate to do and imagine going to work every day to do it. The money won't make you happy; it will slip right through your fingers as you spend it on other things to make up for your misery. Seniors learn to escape into other things, just as every age does. This usually happens when they are disappointed with their life and don't know what to do to change it. Don't get trapped in this long ditch; it takes awhile to crawl out.

TEMPTATIONS OF A SENIOR

Many consider that when one gets old, he or she only exists instead of having a life. Others see us as has-beens, dried up and dead. Some never understand that we still have goals and dreams. They act as if our lives are over so there's nothing to look forward to or expect. How wrong they are!

These last years can be the most important ones of our lives! We are the ones who determine whether we are really living or simply existing. Our days can still be a challenge; we can still reach for that challenge and have fulfilled lives.

Where are you in the plan for your life? Do you sit around, waiting to see what will happen next or do you make something happen? You can, you know. You don't have to wait for someone else to do something, what's stopping you? Get in on the action – refuse to be on the sideline of life, watching it go by day after day.

What did you do to make the past more interesting? Maybe you were a success or maybe you failed. None of that has anything to do with the now of your life. You don't have to be a wallflower; get in there and do whatever you can to make life better! Don't wait for others to lead the way. Why don't you take the lead? You can, you know.

So you're tempted to join an art class? Go ahead, why not? What do you have to lose? Look what you have to gain! You could turn those empty, non-rewarding hours into minutes of excitement! Imagine the time when you share your first painting with others! None will believe that you could make such a beautiful contribution! Work at it; your paintings will become even more beautiful and who knows what the results will be? You might be able to sell them. If this is not possible, think what a personal gift you can give to loved ones! What could top a gift of your very own painting? Let it happen! Stop saying, "I could never do that." How do you know unless you try. Whatever you are considering, at least try; then you will know for sure. If you believe you can't, then go on to an item where you believe that you can.

You would like to go to the flower-arranging class but you're afraid of what others might say? They might even laugh at you? Let them; who cares what someone else might do or think! YOU might make the most beautiful arrangements ever. Some would be so jealous but they would never tell you. Many might make fun of your going to any kind of class at your age. The truth might be that they wish they had the nerve to sign up for that thing they've always wanted to do. Instead of allowing their mocking words to get to you, encourage them to follow their own dreams and learn something new. Learning can be a very exciting thing! I wish every senior citizen could or would go to classes to learn to do what they've always wanted to do! They need to know how wonderful a challenge can be! When you do something you've dreamed of doing, there's nothing like it!

Also, it isn't against the law for you to have fun! You don't have to sit home constantly, staring at the television. Get out, go to dinner with a friend (male or female), go to movies or shows at the local 'little theater'. You might enjoy the musicals, the up-beat tempo. "Homecomings" at churches are a lot of fun. All-day gospel sings give us a terrific day with wall-to-wall food and uplifting music. We might see people we haven't seen in years! Just the fun of being out in life can be exciting! Go ahead, you might enjoy it!

BISCUITS FILLED WITH LOVE

I was in Tampa, Florida to see my new great-granddaughter. Being a grandmother of 13, this GREAT- grandchild business was a new experience for me.

Finding new mother and baby doing great, I settled in for a short visit with my daughter and son-in-law. Having some time with their two young sons was icing on the cake!

During the visit, my grandson Gabriel asked, "Grandma, would you make us some REAL biscuits?" Since cooking and baking is one of my hobbies, I was glad to comply with this request. They always enjoy the dishes I make, which gives them something new and a break for my busy daughter.

As I listened to their raves over my biscuits, my daughter Joy suggested, "Mom, why couldn't you make several batches of biscuits and put them in the freezer? That way, we could have your biscuits whenever we want."

I got busy on that project the next day as I placed dozens of biscuits in a freezer container, using wax paper between layers. Because of this idea, months later I was still basking in their compliments on the biscuits.

The opportunity to show my love, which my daughter and her family enjoyed later in the form of Grandma's biscuits, delighted me. The idea wasn't mine, but I CAN share it with grandmothers across the country. I'm sure grandchildren everywhere would love to have some "real" biscuits!

WHY AM I THE ONLY 70-SOMETHING IN VICTORIA'S SECRET?

I didn't understand it. When I mentioned to a friend that I planned to go to Victoria's Secret, she put her coffee cup down abruptly and stared at me as if I had just landed from another planet. I was explaining why we couldn't meet for lunch the next day. As I reviewed our conversation, I saw the cause of her reaction.

SHE probably thinks that Victoria's Secret is only for 20-year-olds. Wrong! Don't they have beautiful lacy things in there for females? Okay, I'm a female; I can go in if I want! (I decided not to tell her that I go there fairly often.) Don't they sell wonderful perfumes? Just because I'm in my 70s, does that mean I can't smell good? I enjoy smelling good; I use perfume just for ME and it makes my day better. There's nothing worse than a bad-smelling day!

As for the gorgeous undies, who says I don't need lacy underwear? I like pretty things now as much as I did in my 20s, 30s, 40s 50s and 60s. Must I stop now, in my 70s, and start getting those rough knit bloomers that go down to my knees? No thanks! I'm still very much a woman and my preference for lacy underwear and yummy perfume didn't fade when I got on Medicare. So I'm not the 34-24-34 I was awhile back (I won't say how far back), I'm not too bad; a size 10 (or less) who can still strut. You didn't know a 70-something can strut? You haven't learned much, have you? I stand up straight, so everything falls (oops, wrong word!) IS in place. Tummy in, shoulders up and back, head high. You will find that puts a different shape to things.

If I want to go to Victoria's Secret, who's to stop me? If you want to stare at the soap operas and whine because the kids don't call, you can, but get this: I'm not wasting my time doing that. I've already lived most of the soap operas and the kids have their own lives to live, just as I do.

No one sees the lacy stuff? I DO! I know it's there under the proper suit I'm wearing. I find myself smiling when I remember my beautiful underwear. (It doesn't take much to entertain me.) It's as if I have a secret of my own. Let everyone wonder why I'm smiling!

Who cares what everyone thinks? Are they paying my bills? I don't have to share my perfume or show them my lacy underwear. Way to go, Granny!

CHOOSE TO BE HAPPY

Are you aware that you can choose to be happy? We often allow circumstances to knock us down and sometimes out, but we don't have to stay there. It is possible for us to use our determination and begin to enjoy a life of happiness. Too often we are blown to and fro in the winds of strife; we never know from one minute to the next what to expect. The truth is, we usually get what we expect. Sometimes we even make statements to that effect, never realizing the power of our words.

We go around saying, "My life is so messed up; I'll never get out of this rut!" Sure enough, we stay in that rut for days or weeks, months or years. It is up to us to decide that we can change the situation so that we enjoy more happiness in our lives. We must also learn that we can't change anyone; we might be the ones who need to change – in our attitude if nothing else.

Our decision to enjoy being happy will bring us the opportunities to do so. Life was not meant to be a difficult wrangle every day, always fussing and fuming with someone in our circle. We can be more aggressive concerning those happy moments; they are not going to come to us until we decide to reach for them. Sometimes we have to make a choice, either to continue to spin our wheels in the ditch of despair or crawl up higher on a level where life can be more exciting and challenging.

YOU are the one responsible for your happiness, not anyone else. We always blame others for our unhappiness but the truth is that it's not up to them. It's up to us. After spending years in depression, you can bet that I'm going to do all I can to stay where I am. I'm so glad to report that where I am is that I have learned to appreciate the little things often overlooked in the past. It's has given me a whole new outlook on life.

Listening to hundreds of birds singing at dawn gives me a new gratitude for nature. Seeing the beautiful sunset brings a smile plus a feeling of awe. Seeing dew on a spider web that has turned into a pattern of diamonds with the morning sun. I choose to see the beauty around me; this makes me smile. I know about the ugly but I choose not to dwell on it. Beauty uplifts me; ugly drags me down. It's our choice.

Have you ever tried to smile and be down and out at the same time? I'm not sure it's possible. A smile not only transforms our faces but also brings a certain happiness to us.

Years ago my late husband and I were driving from Florida to California. He loved to travel but was not the most fun person to be with on a long trip. During this vacation, however, I learned something that has affected my life since. I learned the power of a smile.

As my husband slowed to make a left turn, I noticed a car at the stop sign, preparing to turn right. Our turn brought us near that car and I glanced at the woman driver. She looked directly at me and gave me the most beautiful smile. Words cannot express how that smile affected me. It was the nicest thing that happened that day, possibly on that whole trip!

Imagine riding thousands of miles, longing for a quiet place of tranquility and you might be surprised that I found myself smiling back at that lady! I was tired and needed a break-stop but there I was, smiling! I could hardly believe the happiness that flooded my being! What a great lesson for me; I think often of that wonderful experience.

Since then I have learned more about the power of a smile. Recently, while walking toward an elderly lady in the cardiac care unit, I noticed that she looked as if she carried the weight of the world. I could imagine her concern for a loved one. I smiled and spoke to her and the transformation was amazing! Her face lit up as she returned my smile.

I practice this picker-upper wherever I go. Such a simple thing to bring gladness to others! It doesn't cost any money; you only need the desire to brighten the day for someone else. At the same time, your day is better as they return that smile.

As one who speaks and/or sings for various groups, I am often surprised to see many frowns in the audience. That is my signal to try my "smile therapy" and it always works! From another angle, one friend said she didn't like to sit in the congregation of her church and look at all the frowns in the choir! Surely, we should see some joy on these faces! If not, some have more growing to do.

These observations confirm the power of a smile. Others notice us in a negative way when we frown and will remember us when we smile. Our faces show a lot of our personality, so remember, someone is always looking!

What a gift we can give each other, sharing the joy of being alive as we practice the therapy and power of a smile! I suggest that we look for an opportunity to smile at someone and notice the difference it will make in our lives.

We will experience more happiness from this simple practice, yet it is not an earth-shaking event. It will shape our lives in a different mold; no more will we walk around with a look of misery on our faces. This expression makes others want to avoid us.

Start smiling and see how your life changes. You will be amazed at the difference it makes, not only for you but also for others.

RISING ABOVE DISAPPOINTMENTS

Everyone has experienced disappointments, either in situations, people or personal relationships. If you've breathing, it is possible you might face disappointment today. So what? We can learn to recognize these times as opportunities to grow. We don't become who we are overnight. Because of the tests in our lives, we can grow more mature and be better able to face the days to come. I can truthfully say that if I hadn't had the traumatic times, I never would have gained the strength to face other problems that came up. We can learn to use the stumbling blocks as stepping stones toward a better life.

Just as a baby can't walk the first time he tries, so are we to learn by doing. Each time we get up again, after being knocked down by another of life's blows, we will have a bit less wobble; soon we will be able to stand and go forward. The secret is in getting up again; don't stay down when you fall, but scramble around until you are on your feet again and then continue on your journey.

There are seniors today who are still holding a grudge toward someone who hurt their feelings in the 1940s. Isn't that a terrible waste of time, not to have enjoyed life to the fullest all those years? To allow some little spot to put a blur on our lives is worse than silly; it's stupid!

Each of us probably has sincere reasons to despise several people of our past. The point is that by hanging onto your hurt, you're not causing any pain to them, but you are causing damage to yourself! You're more intent on revenge and you forget your potential. Hanging onto your grudge can cause you to be less than you were meant to be! No one is doing this to you; you're doing it to yourself!

Believe me, your future will be determined by your thoughts of the past! When you waste your brain power on negative thoughts, that's what will be brought into your life! Negative gets you nowhere! You can stay on that road or you can learn to toss away the hurts of the past and go on toward a terrific future. The past is gone; let it go and start thinking of today. You won't have it again, so why throw it away?

Unless you change your attitude regarding the past, you will find yourself struggling from day to day, dreading all of them, and never having the joy of life. Stop and realize what you are doing to yourself! Life is to be lived instead of dreading the next day. You can't know how priceless each day is until you learn to crawl over your disappointments and allow positive thoughts to keep you on track.

Are we going to continue being wimps and let the situations in our lives bring us down? This isn't necessary, you know; we can see that those things aren't really as important as we thought. Nothing is worth throwing our lives away! Stand up and smell the roses instead of keeping your head in the sand!

If you can't forgive and forget, ask God to help you. He forgives your mistakes when you forgive others. So what is it going to be? Will you toss this one life away because of someone else's actions or words? Can't you see how useless that worn path is? Get a new start and be all you can be!

Today is the day to begin a new life! When you accomplish this, you will wonder why you wasted so many years!

TO WORK OR NOT TO WORK

There are thousands of seniors in the work force. These men and women make a terrific contribution to their companies, and it would be a loss to do without them.

This is a decision that each of us make: to work or not to work. When we have worked many years and reach the age of retirement, many want to take it easy as they grow older. Others prefer to stay busy as long as possible, enjoying the practice of going to work in the world of accomplishment. It can be an important factor in our lives, just having a reason to get up. After a few weeks or months, retirement often gets to be a bore. Days become empty for those who formerly had a specific goal for the day.

It is easy to become listless, even lazy, when we have nothing to do but sit around all day. In this manner we are throwing away our days and our lives. That's why it is very important to have a dream to reach for, maybe now we can reach for the dreams of our youth. Why not? We won't know unless we try!

If we don't want a regular job, we can volunteer to serve at hundreds of places and help others at the same time. It can be extremely rewarding to do special things that fill the needs of certain groups. It might take such little effort to do a really big thing!

Maybe we can use our expertise in specific jobs to accomplish big things. Regardless of our experience, we can fill the need for that special something that we can do. The joy of helping others is a terrific thing. To us it might seem a small thing but to the recipients it might be a huge thing!

Instead of sitting home doing nothing, or throwing away our days, we can volunteer to help various groups in whatever way we are capable of doing. These organizations are sometimes desperate for help such as ours.

YOU CAN'T CHANGE
WHAT YOU TOLERATE

There are always certain things we don't like, especially when they happen to us. As long as we do nothing many of those things will continue, thus bringing us more pain or disappointment. In trying to keep the peace, we often carry it too far as we tolerate bad behavior in others.

Usually we give up and decide that we can't change anyone and this is very true much of the time. We might not change the actions of others, but we don't have to be a part of it or even be near it. Sometimes, because of our closeness, we seem to be part of it. Many times we stand with someone who is not pleasing. We smile and try not to rock the boat. What we are really doing to those looking on is showing that we approve of certain acts and we become a part of the action.

This can be detrimental to our lives and we need to recognize those situations where we should not participate and seem to be part of the overall action.

We will learn that as long as we tolerate something, we will never change it, whether it be an action or person. We know those who are devious as they lie or take things that are not theirs. We look on and sigh our objection but the activity continues and sometimes gets worse. Either we get away from it or let our feelings be known. As long as we say or do nothing, then nothing will change. If it is something we can do something about, do it! Many, regardless of age, still need to learn the meaning of right and wrong; we don't hear a lot about that these days.

When we were growing up, however, that was one of the main subjects we heard from our parents.

Seniors can be as sly as any teenager. Don't believe that because one has silver hair, that person is always trustworthy. It is a painful lesson but one we learn time after time. Most of the time, we want to believe the best about someone. This is good but can also bring us another disappointing experience.

I DIDN'T STOP BEING A WOMAN WHEN I GOT ON MEDICARE!

I have a saying that I repeat more and more often: 'people are strange'. This category is overflowing and yet I find circumstances that fit only in that space. Take an older woman, for example. Many believe that we're just sitting around, sometimes rocking gently in our rockers, but mostly just waiting to die. Wrong!

Understand, this is not the thoughts of only young people but possibly the ideas of our peers. Do you think that teenagers are the only ones who have 'peer groups'? Wrong again! Many, especially males, believe that a silver-haired lady is handy only for baking goodies. This shallowness often causes them to miss out on the blessings of life. Though this idea might apply to a few, most women enjoy being a woman long after they get on Medicare.

None of us invented sex; God did. He meant it to be not only a way to 'be fruitful and multiply' but also a pleasure for us to enjoy in marriage. Certainly many have enjoyed this act in and out of marriage. "It takes all kinds" is one of the old sayings my mother had; I'm glad she didn't learn just what 'all kinds' include. Though I've lived a lot, I'm still shocked at some of the kinds I see; I'm sure my mother would have been speechless.

Many single seniors are constantly looking for a mate, often for the wrong reason. Whether we like it or not, there are those who are devious, including men and women. Many women seek financial security and will grab the most convenient male who might provide it. She doesn't stop to think of the price she might pay for that security. She can have every material item available but still have emotional needs that aren't met. If she is beautiful, or even good looking, she might be the 'trophy' some men need to show off, believing this makes them more of a man. This might be the only category she fills.

Many seniors need someone who will 'take care of them' as they get older. Just as children might choose not to attend to a needy parent, a mate might also prefer not to take care of a spouse. Many have a wedding without a marriage. Remember that marriage does not always provide the answer to our needs. Choosing the wrong mate might bring on more problems than we can handle at out age.

Marriage should involve love, trust and respect but all too often there is a lack of some or all of these. When this happens, you become roommates instead of mates. This is a sad situation to experience. As an older person, there might not be any place you can go to escape your unhappiness. If there is a place, you might be better off to go there; you would at least have peace of mind as to who you are. You must learn not to judge others and it is possible to come to the answer that only they are responsible for their actions. It really is between them and God, though we should pray for them to see the error of their ways. This will help us rise above the situation, whether we have to stay or can go on with our lives at another location.

It takes a lot of courage to pull up our roots and start over but it can be done. It is important to keep our eyes on the goal we have chosen – don't be sidetracked by other things. Decide what our aim is and stick with it!

Don't have the attitude that you won't be able to do something; this is only proven as you fail. Know that you can succeed and try again! The frame of mind makes all the difference!

YOU'RE NEVER TOO OLD TO LEARN

School. That word strikes near-terror in the minds of many. For others it means excitement, fun, challenge and the joy of learning new things.

Years ago, those who attended college were usually planning to teach in some field of education. Now you can prepare for any career by getting a college degree.

One is bedazzled by the classes listed in college brochures, everything from cake decorating and bread baking to creative writing and tole painting. There are many opportunities for those who have the desire and time to meet the challenge of their abilities. This is especially true of the senior citizen who returns to the classroom.

For those whose children have grown and gone, time might hang heavy on their hands. No longer is it necessary to do two or three laundries each day, nor cook for a big family. It's often difficult to scramble up enough for one laundry and mealtime sometimes is a forced activity.

Some suffer from the empty nest syndrome; they don't realize that this can be one of the most wonderful times of their lives. Now they can know who they are besides Mom or Dad.

Whatever you like to do, there are classes to help you do it better! These might be found at community colleges, technical schools or adult education classes. You can have more fun than you thought possible!

A new world will open to you. Instead of staying home, wondering why the kids don't call, get out and do something to jazz up your life. Learn what you're capable of doing. You will be amazed at the difference this will make in your life. It might also change your attitude about life.

Not only do you have the time to spend on learning something new, whether for fun or profit, but you will have a fantastic sense of accomplishment. This might be something you've never experienced. Nothing can compare with that feeling! You will be able to face a challenge head on and learn more about yourself at the same time.

There will be many opportunities to apply your new talents (not really new, just not brought out before). You might improve your personal relationships or begin a new career with the knowledge you have gained. Just knowing you have accomplished something is terrific!

Some might not want a new career or even need to do something to earn money. You might have everything possible, but even then you might not be satisfied with your life. I could never just sit and stare at the walls; I would be very unhappy. Idleness allows us to focus on ourselves, which can make our lives miserable. I'm not wasting my time watching the depressing soap operas; I don't want to take on the problems of those people. I am too busy to get depressed; I spent years there and refuse to return. I've grown into a tough lady who refuses to waste more time on negative thinking; life is too short for that.

Another old saying of my mother's was 'an idle mind is the devil's workshop' and that is definitely true. When we have no goals or plans in mind, we focus on our aches and pains as these become our primary thought pattern. We can and often do literally talk ourselves into being sicker than we really are. How can we help it, when we think of nothing else? These negative thoughts will bring you into a deeper rut and only your thoughts and determination will save you. That's why it is beneficial to get our mind on helping others. There are always many whose situations are worse than ours.

Years ago I attended creative writing classes, hoping to improve my writing ability. I was pregnant and had no intention of sitting around the house waiting for the months to pass. When one class ended, I enrolled in another. The months flew by (so did my pregnancy) and my life was changed forever.

When my youngest child was in kindergarten, I enrolled in morning classes at a nearby community college and finally earned an Associate in Arts degree in Journalism. Actually I wanted to major in about four things but finally chose journalism. I have been involved in the writing and publishing field, as well as music, since 1960.

At age 73, I still apply what I learned in those classes to the things I do today. If I hadn't gone back to school, I might still be in the ditch of despair where I lived so many years.

My first book, WHO DO YOU THINK YOU ARE? dealt with self esteem and was published in 1989. Before I went back to school, I felt lower than a worm and realized that many have this deep sense of failure. That same year, at age 58, I recorded ten of the gospel songs I had written. When I was 68, I recorded a CD, singing harmony on five songs someone else wrote as well as five more of my songs.

During the last 30 years, I've had dozens of freelance articles published in regional, national and international publications. I wrote a newspaper column, ENCOURAGEMENT FOR TODAY, for several years. I edited and published a quarterly newsletter, LIVING WITH HOPE, for 3 years, using the manuscripts of people from around the globe. I wrote and produced a radio program, ENCOURAGEMENT FOR TODAY'S WOMAN, going from weekly to daily programs. I've spoken to many groups and organizations, offering encouragement to those who simply need someone to tell them, 'You can do it!'

I appreciate the opportunity of going back to school and what it did for me. My life was changed from years of failure and pessimism to an open field of opportunity because I had the courage to enroll in classes I would enjoy! There's nothing like learning something new and there's no age limit on learning. The new sense of discovery concerning myself has given me the courage to eagerly face each day with a sense of expectancy.

I continue freelance writing and keep five or six articles in the mail. I'm always eager to get the mail to see if I've had an article accepted. Every day is exciting! I am working on other books, according to my mood. My second book, THE GOLDEN OLDEN DAYS, told of growing up in the rural Florida Panhandle in the 30s and 40s and the family lifestyle of that time.

I recently began art classes and am amazed at the two things I've done. I want to sew better; I'd like to improve my Spanish and refresh my Italian. I'd also like to learn to play a stringed harp.

If someone else can do it, so can I! Who knows what wonderful things I might do at age 78? I'll see you in class!

LEARNING TO LAUGH

I truly like the joy of discovering new information about anything; I'm always amazed at how much I don't know. One of the most wonderful things I have learned and something that really changed my life, is the ability to laugh. Being able to laugh, a lot and often, is one of life's greatest gifts. Not only does it change the expression on our faces, but also our days, even our lives.

Most of us have things in our lives that make us sad. Some major on these things instead of seeing the good in our days. When we hang around negative thinkers, all we talk about are the wrong aspects of our lives. We're so intent on seeing the bad that we fail to see the good that is there. We constantly replay the painful experiences instead of going forward and making something positive happen. This is not possible while we are dwelling on negatives; we have to learn not to expect several negatives to become a positive. Not until we change our thought patterns will we be able to see anything positive in our lives.

Seniors are as bad as younger people; we hit that replay button and swim constantly against the current. We are pushed here and there in our thought life and end up at the same spot on negative island. When will we learn that we don't have to rehash those painful times? Turn them loose and go on to something better!

You are able to do this when you learn that you are the one who controls your thoughts. When we allow situations to be in control we might as well give up. It is too easy to do this and many suffer because of it. What we need is a little grit and determination that we will control our thoughts, thank you. This is one of the greatest things I have learned in life, that I don't have to think on all those painful situations but can turn my thoughts off them and think about the sunset or some other beautiful thing. Many of us knew how to hit the replay button long before VCRs were available. For years we swam upstream in bitter memories, hounded daily by our past. We don't have to do this!

Look at the days, weeks and years we have thrown away! The best medicine for these gloomy thoughts is that we learn to laugh. We might even learn to laugh at ourselves. There is often humor in many things surrounding us; it is up to us to see it and enjoy a chuckle.

There are those I enjoy being around simply because we laugh a lot together. This is preferable to spending time in the company of someone constantly down and out. Be very careful that they don't drag you down with them. Another saying I grew up with is 'birds of a feather flock together'. If you hang around depressed people it might be contagious. Watch out that you don't adopt the same frame of mind of the company you keep. This of course reminds me of another saying, 'show me the company you keep and I'll tell you who you are.' We surely don't want to spend our lives drowning in sadness. When we are more careful of the 'company we keep', we can assure ourselves of better and brighter days. Of course, if we know someone who is depressed, we should do all we can to help them and keep them in our prayers. Be sure, though, that you can influence them for a happier life and that they don't influence you to join them in their rut of depression.

Make certain that you look for humorous situations or people who make you laugh. Not only will this make you a happier person but also your days will be more wonderful. You will learn how to laugh more by doing it. Sometimes the most simple things can be funny; it doesn't take a famous comic to make us laugh. Life can bring many chuckles and I plan to enjoy every one that I can.

First we have to swing our thoughts off the things that cause us regret. Look forward instead of backward. You will find a new kind of life that will help you to look forward to each day. Try it! Soon you might even learn to laugh about many past things as you toss them where they belong.

I can't emphasize enough how important it is for us to laugh a lot. Look at the terrific cartoons in The Saturday Evening Post and other magazines, read the jokes in Reader's Digest, the silly items in the freebie papers we see. LOOK for an opportunity to chuckle.

Once you learn to laugh at life's situations, at others and yourself, you will be on the road to a life with less tension. When we look for strife we will find it. Each day there are stressful events for all of us but we are ahead of the game when we learn to chuckle and go on. Don't allow bad things to get you down in the dumps. See the funny side of life. Yes, you are the one who allows the negatives to affect your life. Why not also learn how to let the positive things of life be our guide for days of challenge and fulfillment? It's up to you; which would you rather have?

CHOICES WE HAVE TO MAKE

All through life we have to make choices and we make them, some good and some bad, as we go along. At times we don't give enough thought to our decisions and often believe that it is not too important. We can be fooled in that we might have long term consequences from those quick choices of the past.

Though all our decisions affect our lives in one way or another, our decisions as a senior are of great importance. It is sometimes necessary to make choices that will determine our future. It is good when we have a choice. Our present and future will be the result of our choices so we should give time and thought before we choose what to do. It is so important that we should pray about our decision and/or talk with a trusted friend as to what might be best for us and our families. Be careful in your choice of the one to discuss your business; you don't want to hear about it next week from a stranger.

We might need to decide whether to stay in our home after our mates have passed away. Remember, it is for you to decide. What might change that situation is whether you are physically able to take care of yourself. Can you take a shower, dress yourself, do the necessary cooking and all the things involved in running a house? This includes taking out the garbage, getting the full can to the point of pick-up, making sure the bills are paid, writing the checks, doing the laundry and all the other necessary things of living alone. The answer depends on whether or not you can.

If you aren't physically able to do those things, then it will be necessary that you make another decision. This one might involve your children or someone who realizes the importance of what needs to be done. Remember, you don't want to set your house on fire, neither do you want to fall and stay there for days. The condition of your health is the key to the answers you will need at this time.

It is never easy to leave our homes but sometimes, for our own good, it is necessary. There might come a time when we aren't capable of doing the things that have to be done. We might be able to know this, but sometimes we can't understand or see why we need to leave our homes so that our lives might be better. This is a painful situation for all involved but it has to be faced. Those who love us don't want more grief in our lives; we need to listen to the wisdom out there for our benefit.

Sometimes it might be possible for us to have someone live in and take care of us. If we can, and know that we can trust this person, this would be a good answer. Be so very careful, though, in the person of your choice. Many who seem to be good and honest really are not. We will need the opinion of someone else at this point. Making a wrong choice here can cause us to lose too much. Some who pretend to be eager to help might steal our things. Those who would do this are sharp enough to find a way without our knowing anything about it.

If we are to be home-bound, then we might decide to share some of our now un-needed items with those who need them. If we aren't going out a lot, share those clothes, clean of course, with others who can use them. There are too many in need and in our particular situation, we might be a real blessing to others. Why not share, if you don't need the items and you know that others do? I knew one lady who loved sweaters; she had 68 of them and seldom wore any of them. What she didn't see were those who really would have been thankful for even one of those sweaters! The weather got cold in that area and many lives could have been blessed.

We need to discuss with someone we trust all the items of importance in our present lives. As seniors, there are so many details to be decided and it is usually up to us to know when to do this. If we can't, it is best if we have already chosen who we want to make those choices for us, for sooner or later it will have to be done.

Few like to talk about the end of our lives, but that time will come to all of us. As we mention in a later chapter, there will be decisions about our passing, where we want our services to be held and our choice of where we will be put at the proper time. These are decisions we can make while we are still able to do so. That might be more satisfactory than having others decide for us. They need to know our opinions on the subject at hand. Talk about these things while you can because at a later time you might not have any say in it.

In the meantime, while we are mentally and emotionally able, we should make the choices most important to us. Others might not know what we want or even might not care, so take care of these things while you can. In many cases, we have known things to be done that would have caused great hurt had the person known it. We can avoid this as we take care of those things that need to be done. Do it today; don't procrastinate. Never put off until tomorrow what should be done today.

DOWNSIZING OUR LIVES

There comes a time for all of us that we have to bring our lives into a tighter circle, or downsize. This is usually for our good and can often be good for others.

The important thing for us as seniors is to recognize this time in our lives. We downsize and still keep our dignity if we go about it in the right way. We shouldn't mourn our past lives but go on toward the future with a smile and love for our families. They will benefit from our decisions now so why should we regret our being able to help them?

For instance, if we can't drive anymore, why not give our vehicle to that grandson or granddaughter who is working so hard to get through college? It will be a blessing to them as they struggle for their future.

It might be that we decide to sell our homestead so we might move into a senior community or retirement home. Do that if it is best for you. A family member might be interested in buying your property, so ask all of them. You might not be able to share the proceeds of that sale yet, for you still have to live somewhere else. Make the decision that is best for you.

If we own a second home, maybe at the beach or other vacation spot, it might be best if we allow our families to take it for their enjoyment. If you need money from it, tell them so they can decide whether or not they want to buy it. It might be that all of your children could go together and buy it from you, for all your grandchildren and great-grandchildren to enjoy in later years.

We should have all these things worked out while we can. Later on we might not be able to make the decisions or tell others what we want. Again, do it now!

DOES BEING OLD MEAN I CAN'T PAINT MY TOENAILS?

Okay, so I'm nearing my mid-seventies. I am proud to be a mother, grandmother and great-grandmother. I never knew my grandparents so I realize that I missed a lot. The thing is, I don't feel old. As an active senior, I'm having the time of my life!

I'm not a card player and I would die if I had to spend my time waiting for Bingo Night. I'm more for going to the libraries, either to get more books, to have book signings or attend signings. I grab a lot of crossword puzzle books (yes, I do them in ink). I don't have time to watch a lot of television unless I'm on it. I don't care to watch the soap operas; I've already been there and refuse to go back. I like to know what is going on in the world, though that could be depressing if I dwelled on it, which I do not. There are some things I can't change and I accept that.

Thank the Lord for audio books. If and when I reach the point that I can't read, I will get those audio books that are available in libraries and stores.

Years ago, when audio books didn't exist, a friend and I used to read to a blind friend. I felt so sad that he wasn't able to enjoy reading.

I wear the same size dress that I wore 50 years ago, though that has risen and fallen over the years. Yes, I have silver hair – by choice, simply because I like it. Yes, I have a few wrinkles but so what? I know just a bit about arthritis; my BP is perfect as is my cholesterol. Like others my age, I sometimes forget things. What I forget most is that I'm an old person.

Sure, I like to have my hair done, what woman doesn't? My nails grow so fast that I have a time keeping them short enough that I can type my articles or books. I see others with everything painted and polished up, though they are often much younger than I. At my age, am I going out on a limb if I paint my toenails? I understand that this is my decision. It's just that my perception of being a "Grandmother" doesn't include painted nails in golden sandals nor the dangling earrings that I love to wear. I'm not dressed until I use my favorite perfume. Did I get off at the wrong station? Yes, I like to cook and bake and have homemade soup on chilly days, but I don't wear an apron everyday like my Mama did.

The truth is my Mama, and others of her generation, didn't have speaking and/or singing engagements, nor television/radio guest spots, nor bylines or book signings. Her life revolved around her eight children. When she was 60, I thought she was old. Why am I not old at going-on 74? Did I miss some important directions? I will confess that while my five were growing up, I stayed home as much as possible by choice. I thought it was important for them to have me at home when they came in. I enjoyed making a home for them and being a home-maker. My oldest son was a great help with the younger ones; I thank him for that. I'm also glad that I could be an at-home Mama.

I have to admit that the world and life has changed considerably since I was growing up. Some of it I like and much of it I don't; I have no control over so many things. All I am responsible for are my own words and actions. Truthfully, I'm having a terrific time! I enjoy the challenges of each day. I thank God for my good health; I am seldom sick; my health is one of the reasons I can be as active as I am. Sometimes I think that I should be an old lady and be done with it. I suppose I will when the time comes.

Two minutes later, I'll get a terrific idea for an article, or think of some unique way to promote my books (this is the third, with at least two to go). I'll have to live twenty more years so I can learn to use my cell phone. I enjoy getting and sending e-mail. I send those attachments like I know what I'm doing. Then my fax starts making a noise and I know something is about to happen. I love to do instant messaging; it's almost as good as a phone call. Does this mean that I'm techy --- or tacky?

No, I don't skip any of the necessary things in running a home, though I will try to avoid ironing. I suppose the methods have changed so much that I have time for other things. Now I have to bring this one-way conversation to a close. See you later, maybe, but I really don't have time to drink coffee and gossip.

I'd better write down those ideas to write about, otherwise I might forget them. Then I have to make an appointment for a manicure and pedicure. I wonder, should I try that mauve color or a brighter red? No, I think I'd like a softer shade; it seems more appropriate for my age.

I need to make sure I can get my hair done in time for that television guest spot. I want to be a sharp looking old lady! Yes, I believe it is possible.

Then I'll start making supper; my daughter and wonderful son-in-law are coming over with their family. I'm sure that little Eddie knows my voice, even if he is just three months old. I love the way he smiles at me! He's such a happy baby!

We'll have coffee at another time; forget about the gossip.

HAVING PEACE OF MIND

It is hoped that all of us have had peace of mind for many years. We know, however, that many never have that special peace that allows them to fully enjoy their lives.

When we live our days and years in stress and strife, it is difficult to look forward even to tomorrow. One of the most wonderful truths is that we can have this peace so that nothing or no one will be able to knock us down. It can take us several years to attain this peace but our frame of mind will be totally different when we have it.

Personally speaking, I began to have peace of mind when I realized that I should make God an important part of my life. As I grew spiritually, I knew that God should be the center of my life. The strange thing is that we can have peace with God without having the peace of God. Many who sit in church every week are so torn up over situations in their lives that they can hardly sit still in church. They spend all their days trying to work everything out for themselves. They have forgotten that God cares about every detail of our lives; He wants to guide us to the right answers. He can't do that when we aren't listening for his direction. We have to be attuned so we don't miss that guidance that can change our lives.

Especially at our age, we don't need stuff in our lives that keep us upset and sometimes devastated. Some of us do not even know that we don't have to experience these things that bring turmoil in our lives. We can learn how to avoid the things that might bring us down.

By refusing to forgive someone, we will live in a state of anger and bitterness. Remember, this doesn't do any harm to those who have hurt you but it definitely eats away at you like a cancer. These deep feelings, carried around all our lives, can bring on diseases that burden us all our lives. Some of us know that our emotional state affects our state of health. Look around you; many that you see every day are in bad health today because they have carried grudges and have refused to forgive. The sad thing is that in order to be forgiven, we have to forgive. What more incentive do we need? All of us need forgiveness.

The first step to having peace of mind is to get in right standing with God. We often learn the hard way that we need to stop ignoring Him and try to get closer to Him. This is not a book on spiritual things but it is about how to live a fuller life. This is possible only when we allow God in our lives. Any other peace of mind is temporary and false.

There are hundreds of evangelists on television as well as churches on many corners in cities. There's no excuse for not knowing about God. When we grow to the point of wanting to be the ones He sees in us, we have come far. We see our failures but He sees our potential. It is too easy for us to dwell on the negative things on our lives but He knows the positive things about us and wants to help us live those positive, rewarding lives. For a fact, we can't and won't do that until we allow Him in our lives and listen to His directions.

What would you give to have peace of mind? When you have it, you'll never want to lose it again! It won't matter what obstacles come at you, nothing can destroy you. You will stand firm, knowing that you are not alone and that God will guide you through any situation. Why don't you try to gain this priceless gift? Your life will never be the same!

ATTENDING TO LEGAL DETAILS

There are many important legal details that need to be taken care of while we are able to do them. This can be done in a simple fashion, good enough to get the facts to the one we have designated to take care of the details after we're gone. We don't like to discuss this particular subject but we need to realize the importance of doing so. When we ignore these things, we bring more grief on our loved ones. They are confused as to what needs to be done and their mourning will be more painful if we don't take care of these details.

While we are able, we should write down facts that our chosen one will need to know. First of all, it is important that we choose someone we trust totally. Sadly, this is not always easy but we have to choose someone. I'm sure it would be legal to choose someone other than our families if we don't have a loved one we can trust. Someone must be chosen to wrap up the legalities of our lives. We need to decide who this someone is while we are able to do so with a clear mind.

We should write down all our debts, such as credit cards, and make this information known. It could be paid off at a later time but none of us know the time we might leave this world, so write it down. Give names and/or addresses of people you might owe. Make sure your family knows if you have a will (you should have) and who is holding it for you.

Share about your life insurance or other insurance that might benefit your loved ones; the location of these policies should be known.

It is time to clear up all the details of your life; this is not a time to be secretive. Your family needs to know things, especially the person you have chosen to take care of these details. Note the bank accounts, whether checking or savings. These need to have the name of someone you trust on the signature card, along with yours. Also, if necessary, make sure someone might have power of attorney so they can sign your name to documents necessary in the future.

If you have any investments, tell all about them on your informative paper. No one will know if you don't tell them! Whatever money you invested will be lost, or taken over by the state or a stranger, if you don't share the details with your loved ones.

Take care of automobile titles as well as property deeds while you can. You don't have to necessarily tell all this information to everyone. One grandmother signed her home over to her only granddaughter, told her about it, and ended up getting put out of that home and had to rent an apartment for the rest of her life. It is painful to think those things go on but we must be realistic and admit that they do.

We should also make a list of friends to be informed of our passing. The locals will know but most of us might have friends in far away places, which could be in other states or even in other countries. It is simple to list their names and phone numbers, maybe their addresses, so this detail can be completed. Much of this can be done through the mail, if preferable. Otherwise a phone call might be better for those we are closer to; our families will know what to do.

ACCEPTING DEATH AS
PART OF LIFE

All of us know that sooner or later our lives will come to an end. Most of us believe that will be a long way down the road but the truth is that we don't really know.

Most don't like to discuss it; some flatly refuse to accept it, but the time will come when we will die. It is better to accept it as part of living, be realistic about it, and go on to enjoy the days and years we are given.

When we get stubborn and refuse to admit that we will die someday, many facts and lives are affected. W can be immature and cause a great deal of trouble for our loved ones or we can choose to work together with them so their mourning is not extended. They will need to bring closure to their grief and a lot of this will have to do with how we act. It is possible to make everything during this time much less painful for our families. Wouldn't we want to do that?

Just talking about our death doesn't mean we want to die. Most of us are eager to postpone that time but we also realize that it will come to one and all. Be brave about it and do the necessary things to make it easier for your family. Do we want them to suffer? Of course not! Then we must work with them, not against them. They are trying to do their best for us; they could refuse to do even that. What could we do? Nothing! So appreciate your loved ones who are willing to help you face these facts. Remember, it's not fun for them either!

It's better to tell them which funeral home you want, where you want to be buried, even the songs you prefer! Tell them the small details that will be important at some time in the future. If you have a favorite dress or suit that you would want instead of a 'shroud', tell them! Have your spot picked out in the cemetery and make sure others know about it!

You are not being dismal, rather you are being sensible! Clear all the clutter! Let the details be known! You can't imagine the gratitude your loved ones will have because they were given all the facts! It's when they know nothing that more grief fills their lives. When they have to look and search for facts they need to know, it makes life more difficult for them and their families.

Your first decision is the name of the one who will take care of the details. Then you are to work on getting all those details down on paper for that person. Don't rely on your memory or theirs. This can fail us at any age. It is best to write everything down.

Instead of watching those depressing soaps, think of those facts that will at some time be very important to your family. Even if you write down just a few facts each day, that is a beginning and tomorrow you can write down a few more. Soon you will have it finished and it will mean a great deal to someone later. It might be better if you have your signature notarized, just to make it official.

When you have finished this, decide to enjoy these days you have left to live. See the glory of the sunset; listen to the hundreds of birds singing just before daylight. Look at the wildflowers in bloom, representing every color. See the beauty of the full moon, enjoy the twinkling of the stars. You can improve your days by listening to beautiful, soothing music. Review all your blessings and you will be amazed at the number of them. Love your families, which is one of your greatest blessings. Be kind to others and help those who need your help. Forgive those who have hurt you. Carry no grudges with you; you don't need that extra weight on your shoulders. It is important to enjoy your solitude. One can be lonely in a big crowd but solitude is a wonderful gift.

Live your life to the fullest and learn to enjoy the gift each day!

WHY THIS BOOK WAS WRITTEN

As an active senior, I spend a lot of time around other seniors. Some of the things I see make me very glad but some things make me sad. I see many who are active in many pursuits, eager to do and be all they can.

It hurts me to see seniors spending their days sitting around, literally throwing their lives away. I've seen those who sit all week longing for bingo night. Others are active in volunteer programs or even with a full or part time job. Those who are active seem much happier than those who have nothing to do but watch the television. Eating and sleeping get pretty boring after awhile, with nothing else to do.

There are some who actually sleep their lives away. Many seniors have various types of medications necessary, so we're told, for our health. It's easy to learn which ones will make us drowsy or help us sleep. So goes our days, down the drain. Many of us have an escape; some won't admit it. We go about our daily lives, choosing the way we spend our days. Even at our age, we are not always wise in our choices of things we should or should not do. We have more opportunities to follow our dreams but we often ignore this available time and toss it away on other useless pursuits.

I want to encourage all seniors to be all they can be and not throw their days away. As a 73-year-old, I'm having the time of my life! Being a great-grandmother doesn't keep me from the winner's circle. I can and will do those things I enjoy and experience that reward of accomplishment! I want others to know and accept that they can still succeed in many chosen fields. Being older doesn't mean we are finished! We might have our best days in the future!

Please don't tell yourself, "Now I'm an old person; life is over!" Not so! Move forward and find out! You might be surprised to find wonderful things in store for you. Get the attitude that the best is yet to come! With that mindset, you will be eager for each tomorrow, wanting to know the wonderful things that might happen today!

Remember to thank God for the gift of each day; open your gift with care and discover all that He has planned for you.

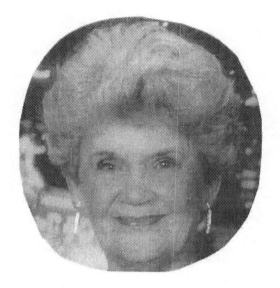

Lura Zerick, author

To contact the author:
Email: Zerick30@yahoo.com

P.O. Box 921
Melbourne, FL 32902